Anti-Inflammatory Eating Plan

50 Healthy Recipes to Change Your Eating Habits

By

Tiara Crocker

© Copyright 2021 by Tiara Crocker - All rights reserved.

This document is geared towards providing exact and reliable information in regards to the topic and issue covered. The publication is sold with the idea that the publisher is not required to render accounting, officially permitted, or otherwise, qualified services. If advice is necessary, legal or professional, a practiced individual in the profession should be ordered.

- From a Declaration of Principles which was accepted and approved equally by a Committee of the American Bar Association and a

Committee of Publishers and Associations.

In no way is it legal to reproduce, duplicate, or transmit any part of this document in either electronic means or in printed format. Recording of this publication is strictly prohibited and any storage of this document is not allowed unless with written permission from the publisher. All rights reserved.

The information provided herein is stated to be truthful and consistent, in that any liability, in terms of inattention or otherwise, by any usage or abuse of any policies, processes, or directions contained within is the solitary and utter responsibility of the recipient reader. Under no circumstances will any legal responsibility or blame be held against the publisher for any reparation, damages, or monetary loss due to the information herein, either directly or indirectly.

Respective authors own all copyrights not held by the publisher.

The information herein is offered for informational purposes solely, and is universal as so. The presentation of the information is without contract or any type of guarantee assurance.

The trademarks that are used are without any consent, and the publication of the trademark is without permission or backing by the trademark owner. All trademarks and brands within this book are for clarifying purposes only and are the owned by the owners themselves, not affiliated with this document.

Table of Contents

Introduction 9
Chapter 1: Breakfast Recipes 10
  1. Scrambled Eggs with Turmeric 11
  2. Smoked Salmon & Poached Eggs on Toast 13
  3. Kale & Pineapple Smoothie 16
  4. Spinach & Feta Frittata 18
  5. Tomato-Arugula Omelets 20
  6. Muffin-Tin Spinach & Mushroom Mini Quiches 22
Chapter 2: Vegetarian & Vegan Recipes 25
  7. Anti-Inflammatory Green Smoothie 26
  8. Golden Milk Overnight Oats 28
  9. Quinoa & Chia Oatmeal Mix 31
  10. Instant Pot Lentil Soup 33
  11. Matcha Green Tea Chia Pudding 35
  12. Kale & Quinoa Salad with Avocado 37
Chapter 3: Poultry & Meat Recipes 39
  13. Baked Turkey Meatballs 40
  14. White Bean and Chicken Chili with Winter Vegetables 42
  15. Chicken Quinoa Fried Rice 44
  16. Sheet-Pan Anti-inflammatory Chicken, Brussels Sprouts & Gnocchi 47

17. Harissa Marinated Chicken Tenders 50

18. Skillet Lemon Chicken & Potatoes with Kale .. 52

Chapter 4: Fish & Seafood Recipes 54

19. Fish Tacos with Broccoli Slaw and Cumin Sour Cream 55

20. Roasted Salmon with Smoky Chickpeas & Greens 57

21. Smoked Salmon Salad with Green Dressing ... 60

22. Greek Roasted Fish with Vegetables 62

23. Garlic Roasted Salmon & Brussels Sprouts 64

24. Provençal Baked Fish with Roasted Potatoes & Mushroom 66

Chapter 5: Soups & Stew Recipes 68

25. Roasted Butternut Squash Apple Soup 69

26. Lemon Chicken Orzo Soup with Kale 71

27. Crockpot Broccoli Turmeric Soup 74

28. Southwest Chicken Soup 76

29. Healthy Slow Cooker Chicken Chili 78

30. Cream of Broccoli Soup 81

Chapter 6: Sauces, Condiments, and Dressings 83

31. Creamy Avocado Lime Dressing 84

32. Coconut Milk Ranch Dressing 85

33. Turmeric-Tahini Dressing 87

34. Super Seed Pesto 88

35. Egg-Free Mayonnaise 89

36. Coconut Butter 90

Chapter 7: Anti-Inflammatory Snacks Recipe 91

37. Frothy Vanilla Turmeric Orange Juice 92

38. Sweet n' Sour Hibiscus Ginger Gelatin Gummies 93

39. Baked Veggie Turmeric Nuggets 95

40. Creamy Pineapple Ginger Slaw 97

41. Turmeric Coconut Flour Muffins Recipe 99

42. Energy Bites with Golden Turmeric 101

43. Ginger Fried Cabbage and Carrots 103

Chapter 8: Dessert recipes 105

44. Hot Chocolate 106

45. Frozen Blueberry Bites 108

46. Anti-Inflammatory Ginger Gummies 109

47. Strawberry-Orange Soft Serve, Sorbet, & Popsicle 111

48. Gluten-Free Vegan Lemon Cake 112

49. Pineapple Upside Down Cake 115

50. Lemon Sorbet 117

Conclusion 119

Introduction

The body's inflammatory response to certain pathogens, such as microbes or chemicals is a natural process of the immune system that prevents the onset of some diseases and protects your health.

When inflammation persists and becomes chronic can produce health issues like arthritis, cancer, heart disease, and Alzheimer.

Studies have shown that one of the most crucial elements to fight inflammation is a proper diet, the one that contains ingredients with plenty of vegetables, whole grains, green protein, nuts, and antioxidants. These are called anti-inflammatory foods due to they can lower the possibilities of having inflammation.

Chapter 1: Breakfast Recipes

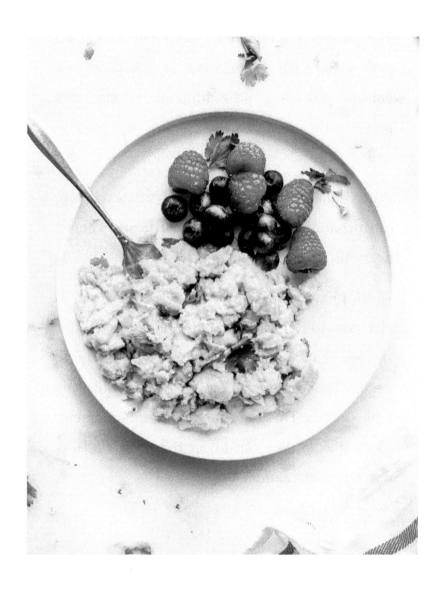

1. Scrambled Eggs with Turmeric

(Ready in about: 15 minutes | Serving: 4 | Difficulty level: Easy)

Nutritional value per serving: Kcal: 187| Fat: 9 g | Net Carb: 27 g | Protein: 8 g

Ingredients

- Olive oil: 2 teaspoons
- Greens Pesto: 1 tablespoon
- 3 organic eggs
- Turmeric: 1 teaspoon
- Salt: to taste
- Coconut milk/cream: 2 tablespoons
- Baby spinach leaves: 100 g
- Chia seeds: 1 teaspoon

Instructions

1. In a dish, whisk the eggs, turmeric, chia seeds, salt, coconut milk until mixed, then set aside.
2. Place 1 teaspoon of olive oil over low to medium heat into a saucepan.
3. Add the spinach, then gently sauté until wilted for 30 seconds.
4. Take spinach off the heat.
5. Heat a tiny small pan with one teaspoon of olive oil over medium heat.
6. Pour in the egg mixture and whisk gently until the eggs tend to settle and become fluffy.
7. Add the spinach wilted, then fold over.
8. Serve with greens pesto right out of the skillet and enjoy it.

2. Smoked Salmon & Poached Eggs on Toast

(Ready in about: 15 minutes | Serving: 4 | Difficulty level: Hard)

Nutritional value per serving: Kcal: 198| Fat: 13 g| Net Crabs: 5.6 g| Protein: 12.7g

Ingredients

For sesame seeds and soy sauce

- 1/2 avocado, smashed
- Lemon juice: 1/4 teaspoon
- Salt and pepper: to taste
- Smoked salmon: 3.5 ounces
- Scallions: 1 tablespoon, sliced
- Bread toasted: 2 slices
- 2 eggs, poached
- Kikkoman soy sauce
- Microgreens, optional

For everything bagel seasoning with tomato

- 1/2 large avocado
- Bread: 2 slices
- Lemon juice: 1/4 teaspoon
- Smoked salmon: 3.5 ounces
- 2 eggs, poached
- Salt and pepper, to taste
- Tomatoes: 2 thin slices
- Microgreens, optional
- Everything bagel seasoning: 1 teaspoon

Instructions

1. Smash the avocado in a dish. Add a pinch of salt and lemon juice; combine properly, and put aside.
2. Poach your eggs, and toast your bread as the eggs rest in the ice water.
3. Place the avocado on both slices once your bread is toasted, then add the smoked salmon to each piece.
4. Place the poached eggs gently on each of the toast.
5. Add a drop of Kikkoman soy sauce and some crushed pepper; scallion, and microgreen garnish.

3. Kale & Pineapple Smoothie

(Ready in about: 5 minutes | Serving: 1 | Difficulty level: Easy)

Nutritional value per serving: Kcal: 110 | Fat: 18 g | Net Crabs: 8 g | Protein: 15 g

Ingredients

- Chopped kale leaves: 2 cups
- Unsweetened vanilla-flavored nut milk: 3/4 cup
- 1 banana, frozen and cut into bite-size pieces
- Non-fat yogurt: 1/4 cup
- Frozen pineapple pieces: 1/4 cup
- Peanut butter: 2 tablespoons
- Honey: to taste

Instructions

1. Put all ingredients kale, banana, almond milk, yogurt, peanut butter, pineapple, and honey in the blender.
2. Pulse the blender till smooth to achieve the required consistency, add more milk. Enjoy.

4. Spinach & Feta Frittata

(Ready in about: 20 minutes | Serving: 4 | Difficulty level: Easy)

Nutritional value per serving: Kcal: 153 | Fat: 18 g | Net Crabs: 10 g | Protein: 20 g |

Ingredients

- Feta cheese: 1/2 cup
- Olive oil: 1 teaspoon
- 1/2 onion, sliced
- Garlic: 1 teaspoon
- Baby spinach: 454 g
- 4 eggs, large
- Salt and pepper: to taste

Instructions

1. Preheat your grill on medium flame, add the oil in the pan.
2. Add the onion and fry until just golden. Add the spinach and toss for 1-2 minutes, once it starts to wilt. Remove from heat and cool it down.
3. In a bowl, crack the eggs. Add the spinach and onion, then the feta, season according to your taste.
4. Place the frying saucepan back on medium heat and add the mixture. Stir softly with a spatula until you notice like the egg starts to set on the bottom. Turn off the fire, to hold the frittata runny.
5. Place the frying pan for 2-3 minutes under the grill or until the frittata is golden and cooked all the way.
6. Place a plate over the pan and easily but gently switch around to remove the frittata. Serve with a crispy side salad, hot or cold.

5. Tomato-Arugula Omelets

(Ready in about: 25 minutes | Serving: 4 | Difficulty level: Medium)

Nutritional value per serving: Kcal: 150 | Fat: 8 g | Net Crabs: 9 g | Protein: 10 g

Ingredients

- 8 eggs
- Pepper to taste
- Fresh arugula / spinach: 1 cup
- Chopped tomato: 1 cup
- Feta cheese: 1/2 cup
- Olives sliced: 1/4 cup

Instructions

1. Cover an 8-inch non-stick skillet with cooking spray. Place skillet over medium heat.
2. In a medium-sized dish, mix egg and pepper. Drop a fifth of the mixture into the prepared skillet. Stir the eggs softly yet constantly with a wooden or plastic spatula right away until the mixture resembles tiny fried eggs covered by liquid egg. Avoid stirring — Cook for longer than 30-50 seconds, or until the egg is set but still shiny.
3. Sprinkle over the egg with some of the arugula, some onion, some of the cheese, and some olives. Lift and fold the other half of the egg over the eggs, using a spatula. Add omelet to a serving tray.

6. Muffin-Tin Spinach & Mushroom Mini Quiches

(Ready in about: 1 hour and 5minutes | Serving: 6 | Difficulty level: Hard)

Nutritional value per serving: Kcal: 240| Fat: 15 g| Net Crabs: 8 g| Protein: 9 g

Ingredients

- Eight large eggs
- Olive oil: 2 teaspoons
- Wild mushrooms: 8 ounces, sliced
- Sliced onion: 1 cup
- Minced garlic: 1 tablespoon
- Minced fresh thyme: 2 teaspoons
- Fresh spinach: 5 ounces, chopped
- Milk: 2/3 cup
- Dijon mustard: 2 teaspoons
- Salt: to taste
- Gruyere cheese: 3/4 cup
- Pepper: to taste

Instructions

1. Preheat oven to 325 °F. Heats the oil over medium flame in a non-stick pan.
2. Place mushrooms in an even layer; fry, untouched, for around 4 minutes until browned on the rim. Stir and proceed to cook for about 5 minutes, stirring regularly until browned all over.

3. Add onion; stirring regularly, around 4 minutes, before they begin to soften.
4. Add the garlic and thyme; roast, stirring, for about 2 minutes, until fragrant. Transfer spinach; cook for around 2 minutes, stirring continuously, until only wilted. Turn heat off.
5. In a large bowl, whisk in the eggs, milk, Dijon, salt, and pepper. Stir in mushroom mixture and cheese.
6. Cover with cooking spray, a regular 12-cup muffin tray. Divide the mixture between the cups. Bake uncovered for around 30 minutes until puffed and finished.
7. Remove from the tray and serve warm.

Chapter 2: Vegetarian & Vegan Recipes

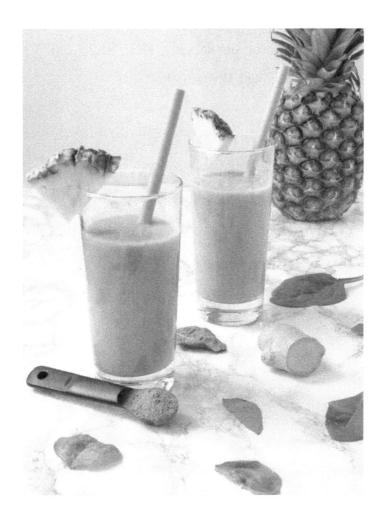

7. Anti-Inflammatory Green Smoothie

(Ready in about: 10 minutes | Serving: 2 | Difficulty level: Easy)

Nutritional value per serving: Kcal: 84.2 | Fat: 3.3 g | Net Carb: 6 g| Protein: 9 g

Ingredients

- Frozen pineapple: 1/2 cup
- Spinach: 2 cups
- Unsweetened vanilla soy milk: 1 cup
- 1/2 frozen banana
- Ginger: 1/4 teaspoon, grated
- Chia seeds: 1 tablespoon

Instructions

1. Put all ingredients in a food blender.
2. Pulse it on high until smooth and creamy.
3. Enjoy.

8. Golden Milk Overnight Oats

(Ready in about: 20 minutes and overnight | Serving: 2 | Difficulty level: Easy)

Nutritional value per serving: Kcal: 195 | Fat: 10 g | Net Crabs: 10 g | Protein: 8 g

Ingredients

For golden milk

- Turmeric: 1/2 teaspoon
- Coconut milk: 1 cup
- Cinnamon: 1/4 teaspoon
- Cardamom: 1/4 teaspoon
- Black pepper: 1/8 teaspoon
- Coconut oil: 1/2 tablespoon
- Ginger: 1/4 teaspoon
- Honey, to taste

For the oats

- Chia seeds: 1 and 1/2 tablespoon
- Steel-cut oats: 1/2 cup

Optional

- Collagen peptides
- Blueberries
- Protein powder
- Nut butter

Instructions

1. Whisk together spices and milk until warm in a small saucepan over low-medium heat.
2. Add the coconut oil and honey. When the honey is dissolved, don't let the mixture get boiling. Remove from the heat the saucepan and allow it to cool for 10 minutes.
3. Add chia seeds, oats, and optional add-ins in a mason jar. Pour a cooled mixture of golden milk into a pot and cover tightly with a lid.
4. Shake the jar until the ingredients have mixed thoroughly before serving. Store in the fridge for 6-8 hours.
5. Serve with coconut flakes, fresh fruit, sprinkle with cinnamon.
6. Enjoy.

9. Quinoa & Chia Oatmeal Mix

(Ready in about: 10 minutes | Serving: 12 | Difficulty level: Easy)

Nutritional value per serving: Kcal: 194 | Fat: 10 g | Net Crabs: 22 g | Fiber: 6 g

Ingredients

- Quinoa: 1 cup
- Rolled oats: 2 cups
- Dried fruit: 1 cup
- Barley flakes: 1 cup
- Chia seeds: 1/2 tablespoon
- Salt: 3/4 cup
- Ground cinnamon: 1 teaspoon

Instructions

1. Combine nuts, barley flakes, dried fruit, Quinoa, salt, and cinnamon in an airtight jar to create the hot cereal dry mix.
2. To produce one serving of hot cereal: add 1/3 of a cup of quinoa and dry mixture of chia oatmeal in a tiny saucepan with milk or water. Let it simmer.
3. Reduce heat, cover, and boil, frequently stirring for 15 minutes until thickened. Let wait for 5 minutes, covered up.
4. If needed, stir in a sweetener, and finish it with dried fruits or nuts.

10. Instant Pot Lentil Soup

(Ready in about: 40 minutes | Serving: 6 | Difficulty level: Medium)

Nutritional value per serving: 305 Kcal | Fat 5.5 g | Net Crabs 7.5 g | Protein 18 g

Ingredients

- Low-sodium vegetable broth: 6 cups
- Olive oil: 2 tablespoons
- Chopped carrots: 1 cup
- Chopped turnip: 1 cup
- Chopped yellow onion: 1 cup
- Thyme: 1 tablespoon
- Fresh baby spinach: 5 cups
- Brown lentils: 2 cups, washed
- Salt: 3/4 tablespoon
- 3 radishes
- Parsley leaves: 1/4 cup
- Balsamic vinegar: 1 and 1/2 tablespoon

Instructions

1. Pick Sauté setting on a multi-cooker programmable pressure.
2. Choose high temperature and let it preheat.
3. Add one tablespoon of oil in a cooker until it becomes hot. Add carrots, onion, thyme, and turnip.
4. Fry, frequently stirring, for around 5 minutes, until the onion is tender. Stir in stock, salt, and lentils.
5. Select cancel. Let the steam release.
6. Before removing the cover from the cooker, stir in vinegar and spinach.
7. Toss the parsley and radishes in a wide bowl with the one tablespoon oil.
8. Put the soup in six bowls, garnish with radish mixture.

11. Matcha Green Tea Chia Pudding

(Ready in about: 30 minutes | Serving: 4 | Difficulty level: Medium)

Nutritional value per serving: Kcal: 155 | Fat: 8 g | Net Crabs: 16 g | Protein: 4 g

Ingredients

- Maple syrup: 2 tablespoons
- Almond milk: 2 cups
- Raspberries: 1 cup
- Vanilla extract: 1 teaspoon
- Chia seeds: 6 tablespoons
- Matcha powder: 1 teaspoon
- Blueberries: 1 cup

Instruction

1. In a mixer, whisk together the matcha, milk, sweetener, and vanilla until creamy.
2. let this liquid pour on chia seeds. Mix it well. Stir again for the next 15 minutes, every 2 minutes. Allow the mixture to stay in the fridge for at least 1 hour or overnight.
3. After taking out from the refrigerator, serve with fresh berries.

12. Kale & Quinoa Salad with Avocado

(Ready in about: 35 minutes | Serving: 2 | Difficulty level: Easy)

Nutritional value per serving: Kcal: 123 | Fat 10 g | Net Crabs: 20 g | Protein: 13 g

- ¼ cup olive oil
- 2 tablespoons lemon juice
- 1 ½ tablespoon Dijon mustard
- ¾ teaspoon sea salt
- ¼ teaspoon ground black pepper

Instructions

1. In a saucepan, put the quinoa and 1-1/3 cup of water to a boil. Reduce the heat to medium-low, cover, and simmer for around 15 to 20 minutes until the quinoa is tender and the water is absorbed. Set to cool aside.

2. Place the kale in a steamer basket in a saucepan over 1 inch of boiling water. Cover the saucepan with a lid and steam for about 45 seconds until it is hot; move to a large bowl. Quinoa, avocado, bell pepper, cucumber, red onion, and feta cheese on top of kale.

3. In a bowl, whisk together the olive oil, lemon juice, Dijon mustard, sea salt, and black pepper until the oil emulsifies into the dressing; pour the salad over.

Chapter 3: Poultry & Meat Recipes

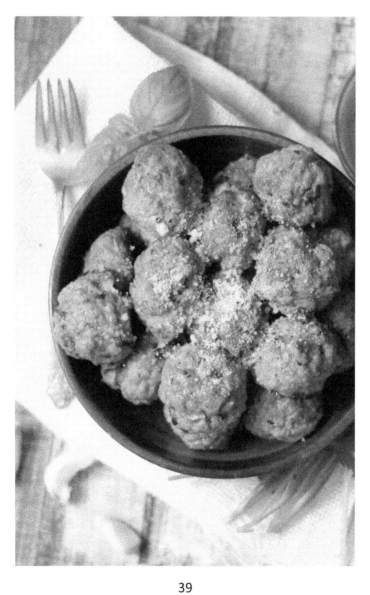

13. Baked Turkey Meatballs

(Ready in about: 40 minutes | Serving: 8 | Difficulty level: Hard)

Nutritional value per serving: Kcal 216 | Fat 3g | Sodium 17mg | Protein 22g | Carbohydrates 32g

Ingredients

- 1 beat egg
- Minced turkey: 454 g
- Grated Parmesan cheese: 1/2 cup
- Fresh breadcrumbs: 1/2 cup
- Chopped parsley: 1 tablespoon
- Milk: 2-3 tablespoons
- Chopped fresh basil: 1/2 tablespoon
- Grated nutmeg: a pinch
- Chopped oregano: 1/2 tablespoon

Instructions

1. Let the oven pre-heat to 350 °F.
2. Put parchment paper on 2 baking sheets.
3. In a big bowl, add the turkey, breadcrumbs, cheese, herbs, egg, nutmeg, cinnamon, pepper, and milk. The amount of milk you can use needs to be changed depending on how dry your bread. The mixture should be moist that it binds together.
4. Roll parts of the meat into roughly 1-inch balls using a teaspoon, and put them onto a baking sheet. You should finish off with 25-30 meatballs.
5. Bake the meatballs for around 30 minutes, frequently rotating, causing the meat to be cooked through and brown gently.

14. White Bean and Chicken Chili with Winter Vegetables

(Ready in about: 30 minutes | Serving: 4 | Difficulty level: Medium)

Nutritional value per serving: Fat 3g | Sodium 17mg | Potassium 50mg | Carbohydrates 32g |

Protein 6g

Ingredients

- 1 seeded jalapeno pepper
- Olive oil: 2 tablespoons
- 1 chopped leek
- 2 minced cloves of garlic
- 1 chopped small onion
- Dried oregano: 1 teaspoon
- Ground cumin: 1 tablespoon
- Crushed red pepper flakes: a pinch
- 1 cup of milk, any sort
- 1 chopped potato

- Chicken /vegetable stock: 3 cups
- Chopped Brussels sprouts: 1 cup
- Cooked and shredded chicken breast: 2 cups
- Can of white beans: 15 ounces

Instructions

1. Placed the skillet over medium heat add olive oil. Add the leek, onion, jalapeno, and cook for around 5 minutes, until the leeks and onion are soft and translucent.
2. Add the spices and garlic to the saucepan, and cook for another minute, stirring.
3. Include the Brussel sprout, potato, white beans, the broth, and the chicken. Simmer for 20 minutes before the bits of potato are soft.
4. Add the milk and cook until it warms up. Serve hot with as needed garnish.

15. Chicken Quinoa Fried Rice

(Ready in about: 35 minutes | Serving: 4 | Difficulty level: Medium)

Nutritional value per serving: Kcal: 425 | Fat: 20 g | Net Crabs: 19 g | Protein: 31 g | Fiber: 5 g

Ingredients

- Boneless skinless chicken thighs: 454 g, cut into 1/2-inch pieces
- Peanut oil plus: 3 tablespoons
- 3 thinly sliced scallions
- Cold cooked quinoa: 2 cups
- 2 beaten eggs
- Diced carrot: 1/2 cup
- Peas: 1/2 cup
- Light soy sauce: 3 tablespoons
- Diced red bell pepper: 1/2 cup
- Toasted sesame oil: 1 teaspoon
- Minced garlic: 2 teaspoons
- Grated fresh ginger: 2 teaspoons

Instructions

1. Heat 1 teaspoon of oil over a high flame in a wok. Add the eggs and cook for around 30 seconds, without stirring, until completely cooked on 1 side. Flip and cook for about 15 seconds, until just cooked completely. Move them to a cutting board, and cut them in 1/2-inch pieces.
2. Add one spoonful of oil to the pan and ginger, scallions, garlic, fry, stirring, for around 30 seconds, until the scallions have softened. Add chicken and cook for 1 minute, stirring.

3. Add carrot, bell pepper, and peas; cook for almost 5 minutes, stirring, until soft. Move all this to a large tray.
4. Add 1 tablespoon of oil to the saucepan and then add quinoa and stir for 1-2 minutes until hot. Stirring constantly.
5. Add the eggs, meat, and vegetables again back into the tub. Add or soy sauce and mix well.
6. Serve sliced with sesame seed.

16. Sheet-Pan Anti-inflammatory Chicken, Brussels Sprouts & Gnocchi

(Ready in about: 40 minutes | Serving: 4 | Difficulty level: Easy)

Nutritional value per serving: Kcal: 304 | Fat: 20.9g | Net Crabs: 23.6g | Protein: 19.9 g

Ingredients

- 4 pieces of boneless skinless chicken thighs
- Olive oil: 4 tablespoons
- 2 minced cloves of garlic minced
- Ground pepper: 1/2 teaspoon
- Chopped fresh oregano: 2 tablespoons
- 454 g of Brussels sprouts
- Sliced red onion: 1 cup
- Cherry tomatoes: 1 cup
- Package gnocchi: 1170 g
- Red-wine vinegar: 1 tablespoon
- Salt: 1/4 teaspoon

Instructions

1. let the oven preheat to 450 °F.
2. In a big bowl, whisk together two teaspoons of oil, 1 tablespoon of oregano, 1/2 the garlic, 1/4 teaspoon of pepper, and 1/8 teaspoon salt.
3. Add onion, Brussels sprouts, and gnocchi; stir to cover. Place over a broad baking sheet.

4. In the large bowl, add 1 tablespoon of oil, the remaining one tablespoon of oregano, the remaining garlic, 1/4 teaspoon of pepper, and 1/8 teaspoon of salt.
5. Add the chicken to cover, and toss. Mix the chicken in a combination of vegetables — Cook for 10 minutes.
6. Take the tomatoes from the oven, and mix to combine. Continue to roast until the sprouts in Brussels are soft, and the chicken is cooked through about 10 more minutes.
7. In the vegetable mixture, whisk in the vinegar and the remaining one tablespoon of oil.

17. Harissa Marinated Chicken Tenders

(Ready in about: 40 minutes | Serving: 4 | Difficulty level: Medium)

Nutritional value per serving: Kcal: 206 | Fat: 18.7g | Net Crabs: 21.0 g | Protein: 20.1 g

Ingredients

- Plain Greek yogurt: 1/4 cup
- Harissa paste: 2 tablespoons
- Boneless, skinless chicken: 2 pounds (18-24 tenders)
- Dry white wine: 1/4 cup

Instructions

1. Put Harissa, yogurt, and wine together. In a baking dish, put the chicken tenders, and cover with the yogurt mixture. Cover with wrap put it in the refrigerator. Marinate for 2 hours or so before midnight.
2. Chicken Cooking: fire up the grill. Take out the chicken from the marinade to make any excess drip away. Put the chicken on the hot grill, and cook on either side for around 5 minutes.
3. Serving ideas: with a side bowl of rice, couscous, quinoa, or in a sandwich. with herbs and sautéed vegetables

18. Skillet Lemon Chicken & Potatoes with Kale

(Ready in about: 50 minutes | Serving: 4 | Difficulty level: Medium)

Nutritional value per serving: Kcal: 347 | Fat: 19.3 g | Net Crabs: 25.6 g | Protein: 24.7g

Ingredients

- Chopped tarragon: 1 tablespoon
- Boneless, skinless chicken thighs: 454 g(trimmed)
- Ground pepper: 1/2 teaspoon
- Olive oil: 3 tablespoons
- Salt: 1/2 teaspoon
- Light chicken broth: 1/2 cup
- Baby kales: 6 cups
- 1 sliced lemon
- 4 cloves of minced garlic
- Baby Yukon gold potatoes: 454 g; halved lengthwise

Instructions

1. Let the oven pre-heat till 400 °F.
2. In a large skillet, heat 1 tablespoon of oil.
3. Sprinkle with 1/4 teaspoon of salt and pepper on chicken. Cook, rotating once, before browning on both sides, a total of about 5 minutes. Move into a tray.
4. Add 1/4 teaspoon of salt and pepper to the pan with the remaining 2 teaspoons of oil, with potatoes.
5. Cook potatoes, cut-side down, for around 3 minutes, until browned. Add lemon, broth, garlic, and tarragon. Bring the chicken back into the pan.
6. Switch the frying pan to the oven.
7. Roast, about 15 minutes, before the chicken is completely cooked and the potatoes are soft.
8. Stir the kale into the mixture and roast for 3-4 minutes until it has wilted.

Chapter 4: Fish & Seafood Recipes

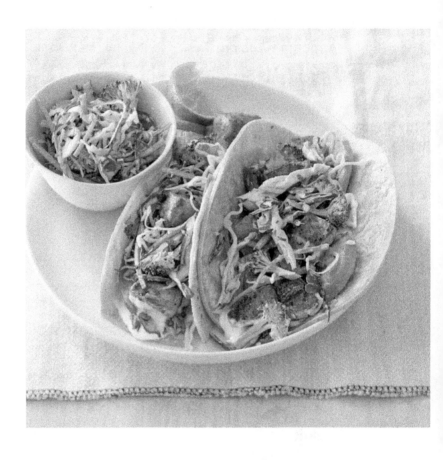

19. Fish Tacos with Broccoli Slaw and Cumin Sour Cream

(Ready in about: 25 minutes | Serving: 4 | Difficulty level: Medium)

Nutritional value per serving: Kcal: 201 | Fat: 14.08 g | Net Crabs 16.78 g | Protein: 20.32 g

Ingredients

- 8 tortillas.
- Frozen fish sticks: 2 10-ounce packages
- 1/2 sliced red onion
- 2 limes, juiced and wedges
- Broccoli: 340 g
- Kosher salt: 1 teaspoon
- Olive oil: 2 tablespoons
- Sour cream: 1/2 cup
- Cilantro: 1 cup
- Ground cumin: 1/2 teaspoon

Instructions

1. According to the direction on the package, cook the fish sticks.
2. Chop broccoli' heads. Peel the stalks and cut them into matchsticks.
3. In a large bowl, add the lime juice, onion, and 3/4 teaspoon of salt., mix and set aside around 10 minutes.
4. Add broccoli stalks and tops, oil, cilantro, and mix.
5. Mix cumin, sour cream, and salt in a small dish. Serve with fish.

20. Roasted Salmon with Smoky Chickpeas & Greens

(Ready in about: 40 minutes | Serving: 4 | Difficulty level: Medium)

Nutritional value per serving: Kcal: 247| Fat: 21.8 g | Net Crabs 23. g| |Protein: 37 g

Ingredients

- Wild salmon: 566 g, cut in 4 pieces
- Chopped kales: 10 cups
- Olive oil: 2 tablespoons
- Salt: 1/2 teaspoon
- Can of chickpeas: 425 g
- Garlic powder: 1/4 teaspoon
- Buttermilk: 1/3 cup
- Mayonnaise: 1/4 cup
- Smoked paprika: 1 tablespoon
- Water: 1/4 cup
- Ground pepper: 1/2 teaspoon
- Chives: 1/4 cup

Instructions

1. let the oven pre-heat until 425 °F and put the racks in the upper third portion, middle of the oven.
2. In a bowl, add 1 spoon of paprika, oil, 1/4 teaspoon of salt.
3. Dry the chickpeas and mix with the paprika blend, put them on a baking sheet, and bake for 1/2 hour on the upper rack.
4. In the food, blender adds puree buttermilk, basil, mayonnaise,1/4 teaspoon of pepper, and garlic powder pulse until creamy. Set it aside.

5. Heat a skillet, add 1 tablespoon of oil over medium flame.
6. Add the kale, cook for 2 minutes. Add water and keep cooking, around 5 minutes until the kale is soft.
7. Remove from flame, and add salt in the dish.
8. Take out the chickpeas from the oven, transfer them to 1 side of the pan. Place the salmon on the other hand, and season with salt and pepper.
9. Bake for 5-8 minutes until the salmon is completely cooked.
10. Top with dressing, herbs, and serve with kale and chickpeas.

21. Smoked Salmon Salad with Green Dressing

(Ready in about: 25 minutes | Serving: 4 | Difficulty level: Medium)

Nutritional value per serving: Kcal: 410 | Fat: 20.1 g | Net Crabs: 26.6 g | Protein: 17. g

Ingredients

- Smoked salmon: 180 g
- Washed green lentils: 1/2 cup
- Yogurt: 1/2 cup
- Parsley: 2 tablespoons
- Salted baby capers: 1 tablespoon
- Chives: 2 tablespoons
- 2 sliced small fennel bulbs
- Tarragon: 1 tablespoon
- Grated lemon rind: 1 teaspoon
- 1/2 onion, sliced
- Baby spinach: 60 g
- Fresh lemon juice: 1 tablespoon

- 1/2 sliced avocado
- Sugar: 1 pinch

Instructions

1. Let the lentils cook for 20 minutes or until soft, in a wide saucepan of boiling water. Then drain.
2. In the meantime, heat a pan on high flame. Spray oil on slices of fennel. Cook per side for 2 minutes, or until soft.
3. In a food processor, pulse the parsley, yogurt, chives, capers, tarragon, and lemon rind until creamy. Season with black pepper.
4. In a bowl, place the sugar, onion, juice, a pinch of salt. Drain after 5 minutes.
5. In a wide bowl, add the lentils, onion, fennel, avocado, spinach. Divide into plates. Put salmon on top. Drizzle with green dressing and fennels.

22. Greek Roasted Fish with Vegetables

(Ready in about: 55 minutes | Serving: 4 | Difficulty level: Medium)

Nutritional value per serving: Kcal: 222 | Fat: 18.6 g | Net Crabs 21.5 g | Protein: 12.9 g

Ingredients

- 4 frozen skinless salmon fillets: 170 g
- 2 red, yellow, orange sweet peppers, cut into rings
- Fingerling potatoes: 454 g
- 5 cloves of chopped garlic
- Cherry tomatoes: 2 cups
- Sea salt: 1/2 teaspoon
- Olive oil: 2 tablespoons
- Black pepper: 1/2 teaspoon
- Pitted halved olives: 1/4 cup
- 1 lemon
- Parsley: 1 and 1/2 cup
- Finely snipped fresh oregano: 1/4 cup

Instructions

1. let the oven preheat to 425 °F.
2. Put the potatoes in a bowl. Drizzle 1 spoon of oil, sprinkle with 1/8 teaspoon of salt and garlic. Mix well, shift to the baking pan, cover with foil. Roast them for half 1 hour.
3. In the meantime, thaw the salmon. Combine the tomatoes, sweet peppers, parsley, oregano, olives, 1/8 teaspoon salt, and pepper in the same bowl. Add 1 tablespoon of oil, mix well.
4. Wash salmon and dry it with paper towels. Sprinkle with 1/4 teaspoon of salt and black pepper.
5. Put sweet pepper over potatoes, and on top of it, salmon. Uncover it and roast for 10 minutes or until salmon starts to flake.
6. Add lemon zest and lemon juice over salmon and vegetables.
7. Serve hot.

23. Garlic Roasted Salmon & Brussels Sprouts

(Ready in about: 45 minutes | Serving: 6 | Difficulty level: Medium)

Nutritional value per serving: Kcal: 334 | Fat: 15.4 g | Net Crabs: 10.3 g | Protein: 33.1 g

Ingredients

- 6 portions of wild salmon fillet: 907 g
- Olive oil: 1/4 cup
- White wine: 3/4 cup
- Oregano: 2 tablespoons
- 14 cloves of garlic
- Salt: 1 tsp.
- Lemon as per choice: Optional
- Black pepper: 3/4 teaspoons

Instructions:

1. Let the oven pre-heat to 450 °F.
2. Take 2 cloves of garlic and mink them. Put them in a bowl 1 tablespoon of oregano, oil, 1/2 teaspoon of salt, and 1/4 teaspoon of pepper.
3. In a roasting pan, halve the remaining garlic and add with Brussels sprouts and 3 tablespoons of seasoned oil.
4. Roast for 15 minutes, stirring only once.
5. Add the wine to the remaining oil blend.
6. Take out from the oven, mix vegetables, and put salmon on top.
7. Sprinkle the wine oil, and salt, pepper, and oregano. Bake for 10 minutes more or until fish is cooked completely.
8. Serve with lemon.

24. Provençal Baked Fish with Roasted Potatoes & Mushroom

(Ready in about: 60 minutes | Serving: 4 | Difficulty level: Hard)

Nutrition facts per serving: Kcal: 276 | Fat: 8.8 g | Net Crabs 25.3 g | Protein: 24.4 g

Ingredients

- Halibut: 397 g, cut into four pieces
- Yukon Gold potatoes cubed: 454 g
- Olive oil: 2 tablespoons
- Salt: 1/4 teaspoon
- Herbs: 1 teaspoon
- Sliced mushrooms: 454 g
- 2 cloves of sliced garlic
- Lemon juice: 4 tablespoons
- Ground pepper: 1/4 teaspoon
- Thyme

Instructions

1. Let the oven heat until 425 °F.
2. Add 1 tablespoon of oil, potatoes, mushroom, pepper, and salt in a bowl.
3. Transfer it to a baking dish, and roast for almost 40 minutes until the vegetables are soft.
4. Stir the vegetables and add garlic.
5. Place fish over it—drizzle with 1 tablespoon of oil, and lemon juice.
6. Sprinkle with herbs bake till fish is flaky for 15 minutes.

Chapter 5: Soups & Stew Recipes

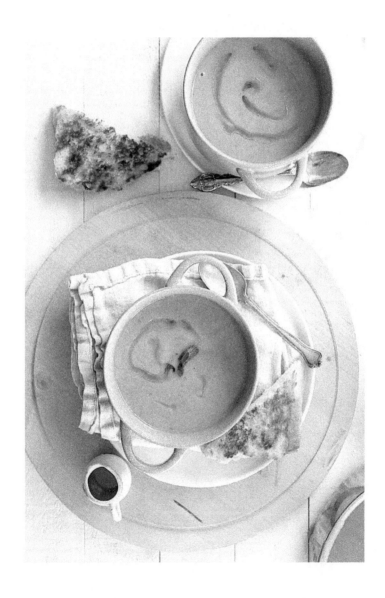

25. Roasted Butternut Squash Apple Soup

(Ready in about: 40 minutes | Serving: 6 | Difficulty level: Medium)

Nutritional value *per serving:* Kcal: 178 | Fat: 10 g | Net Crabs: 15 g | Fiber: 3 g | Protein: 10 g

Ingredients

- Light chicken/ vegetable stock: 3 cups
- Ginger: 1/4 teaspoon
- Olive oil: 4 tablespoons
- Red, sweet apples, chopped: 4 cups
- 1 diced onion
- Chopped butternut squash: 6 cups
- 1 diced celery
- Cinnamon: 1/4 teaspoon
- Salt
- Water: 1 cup
- Pepper
- Nutmeg: 1/4 teaspoon

Instruction:

1. Let the oven pre-heat to 400 °F.
2. Put the squash on a sheet pan and the apples on another sheet pan.
3. Season the squash with 1 and a 1/2 spoonful of olive oil, salt, and pepper, and add only olive oil to apples.
4. Roast the apple and squash for 1/2-hour minutes, until soft.
5. In the meanwhile, cook the remaining 1 and 1/2 spoonful of olive oil over medium flame in a big pan.
6. Sauté the onion and celery until soft. Add pepper and salt to taste.
7. Add stock and let it simmer.
8. When apples and squash are done roasting, add them to the pan along with nutmeg, ginger, and cinnamon.
9. Blend the soup with a blender until creamy.
10. Add salt and pepper according to taste.
11. Serve hot.

26. Lemon Chicken Orzo Soup with Kale

(Ready in about: 40 minutes | Serving: 6 | Difficulty level: Medium)

Nutritional value per serving: Kcal: 245 | Fat: 12 g | Net Crabs 20 g | Protein 12 g

Ingredients

- Chicken broth: 4 cups
- Chicken breasts: 454 g, 1-inch pieces
- Dried oregano: 1 teaspoon
- Olive oil: 2 tablespoons
- Salt: 1 and 1/4 teaspoon
- Diced onions: 2 cups
- 1 bay leaf
- Orzo pasta: 2/3 cup
- Diced celery: 1 cup
- Chopped kales: 4 cups
- 2 cloves of minced garlic
- Diced carrots: 1 cup
- 1 lemon juice and zest
- Black pepper: 3/4 teaspoon

Instructions

1. Heat 1 tablespoon of oil over medium flame in a big pot. Add the chicken, salt, pepper, and 1/2 teaspoon of oregano. Cook for 5 minutes until light brown. Move the chicken to the plate.
2. Add the remaining one spoonful of oil, carrots, onions, celery, and carrots in the same pot.
3. Cook for 5 minutes until the vegetables are tender. Add the bay leaf, garlic, and 1/2 teaspoon oregano. Cook for around 30-60 seconds.

4. Add broth and let it boil over a high flame, adding orzo. Then lower the heat for 5 minutes to let it simmer, cover, and let it cook.
5. Add the chicken and kales and any leftover juices. Continue cooking for 10 minutes until the orzo is soft and the chicken is cooked.
6. Remove from flame. Throw away the bay leaf. Add lemon zest and lemon juice, 3/4 teaspoon, salt, and 1/4 teaspoon of pepper.

27. Crockpot Broccoli Turmeric Soup

(Ready in about: 2 hour and 50 minutes | Serving: 6-8 | Difficulty level: Medium)

Nutritional value per serving: Kcal: 126 | Fat: 7 g | Net Crabs: 11 g | Protein: 7 g

Ingredients

- Stock: 6 cups
- Butter: 2 tablespoons
- Grated ginger: 2 tablespoons
- Broccoli: 8 cups
- Chopped leeks: 4 cups
- Salt: 1 teaspoon
- Black pepper
- Ground turmeric: 1 teaspoon
- Sesame oil: 1 tablespoon

Instructions

1. Heat the butter over medium flame in a big skillet.
2. Add the leeks and let it cook for around 8 minutes until the leeks are completely cooked.
3. Move the leeks with broccoli, ginger, turmeric, sesame oil, salt, and stock to a slow cooker.
4. Cover it, let it cook for 4 hours until broccoli is soft.
5. Blend with a blender.
6. Serve with yogurt and croutons.

28. Southwest Chicken Soup

(Ready in about: 50 minutes | Serving: 4 | Difficulty level: Medium)

Nutritional value per serving| Kcal: 252| Fat: 12 g | Net Crabs: 17g | Protein: 21 g

Ingredients

- Chicken stock: 9 cups
- Chicken breasts: 512 g
- Broccoli florets: 2 and 1/4 cups
- 3 cloves of minced garlic
- Olive oil: 2 tablespoons
- Chopped cabbage: 3 cups
- 1 diced onion
- 63 g of chopped green chilies
- Ground cumin: 1 tablespoon
- Crushed red pepper: 1 teaspoon
- Turmeric: 1/2 teaspoon
- Fire-roasted tomatoes: 308 g
- Carrots: 1.88 cups
- 1 and 1/2 chopped avocados

- <u>Salt</u>
- Pepper

Instructions

1. Placed a big pot over medium flame. Add the onion, olive oil, and garlic. Sauté for 5 minutes.
2. Add chicken breast, diced green chilies, smashed tomatoes, all the spices, chicken broth, and 1 and 1/2 teaspoon of sea salt.
3. Let it boil, lower the flame, and let it simmer for more than 20 minutes tilt the chicken is completely cooked.
4. Take out the chicken and place them to cool off.
5. Add sliced broccoli and cabbage to the pot. Let it simmer until broccoli becomes soft. Shred the chicken and add it back in the pot.
6. Add pepper and salt as required.
7. Serve with diced avocados.

29. Healthy Slow Cooker Chicken Chili

(Ready in about: 3 hour and 10 minutes | Serving: 6 | Difficulty level: Medium)

Nutritional value per serving: Kcal: 223 | Fat 15 g | Net Crabs: 35 g | | Protein: 62 g

Ingredients

- 1 can of undrained, chopped fire-roasted tomatoes
- 1 diced green bell pepper
- 1 diced jalapeño pepper
- Chicken breasts: 2 pounds.
- 1 diced onion
- Chili powder: 1 tablespoon
- Paprika: 1 teaspoon
- 1 can of black beans
- Kosher salt: 1/2 teaspoon
- Ground cumin: 1 and 1/2 teaspoons
- Cayenne: 1/4 teaspoon
- 1 can of diced undrained green chilies
- 1 can of kidney beans

- Light chicken broth:1-2 cups

Instructions

1. In a slow cooker, add diced pepper and onions, and jalapeno.
2. In a small bowl, add cumin, chili powder, paprika, cayenne, and salt and stir well.
3. Take 1/2 of the spice blend, and season the chicken breasts. Put it on onion and peppers in the cooker.
4. Add in the slow cooker with the chilies, tomatoes, and one cup of broth, then add the leftover seasoning.

5. Cook for almost 4 hours on high or 6-7 hours on low.
6. When the cooking time is over, move the chicken breasts from the slow cooker to a board and add the beans to the cooker.
7. Add more broth. If the chili ends up being too thick until you get the consistency you require.
8. Shred the chicken into bits, add the chicken back to slow cooker, and mix season with pepper, salt to your liking.
9. Serve, and eat.

30. Cream of Broccoli Soup

(Ready in about: 30 minutes | Serving: 4 | Difficulty level: Medium)

Nutritional value per serving: Kcal: 151| Fat: 5 g | Net Crabs: 23 g | Protein: 8 g

Ingredients

- Vegetable broth: 3 cups
- Olive oil: 1 tablespoon
- 1 celery stalk, diced
- Broccoli florets: 8 cups
- Salt: 1 teaspoon
- 1 diced onion
- Ground garlic: 1/2 teaspoon
- White pepper: 1/4 teaspoon
- Celery seeds: 1/8 teaspoon
- Cauliflower florets: 4 cups
- Non-dairy milk: 1 cup
- Onion powder: 1/2 teaspoon

Instructions

1. Put a pot over medium flame, and heat the olive oil in it.
2. Stir in the salt, onion, celery, pepper, and cook for 3 minutes until mildly fragrant.
3. Stir in onion powder, garlic powder, cauliflower florets, celery seeds, seven cups of broccoli florets, and vegetable broth. Cover it partially and cook until both types of florets are tender, almost for 10 minutes.
4. Blend the soup in a blender until creamy.
5. Return it to the stockpot once all the soup has been mixed; cut the last cup of broccoli thinly and stir into the soup together with milk.
6. Simmer it, then remove it from the flame, and serve hot.

Chapter 6: Sauces, Condiments, and Dressings

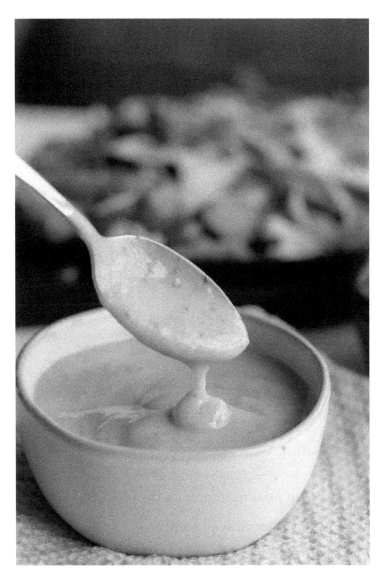

31. Creamy Avocado Lime Dressing

(Ready in about: 10 minutes | Serving: 8-10 | Difficulty level: Easy)

Nutritional value per serving: Kcal: 123 | Fat: 12.3 g | Net Crabs: 4 g | Fiber: 2.6 g | Protein: 0.8 g

Ingredients

- Olive oil: 1/4 cup
- 1 and 1/2 avocados
- Water: 1/4 cup
- Pepper: 1/8 teaspoon
- Crushed garlic; 1/2 teaspoon
- Lime juice: 1/4 cup
- Cilantro: 1/4 cup
- Salt: 1/4 teaspoon
- Cumin: 1/8 teaspoon

Instruction

1. Put all ingredients in the blender.
2. Pulse until well combined.
3. Store or serve right away.

32. Coconut Milk Ranch Dressing

(Ready in about: 10 minutes | Serving: 8-10 | Difficulty level: Easy)

Nutritional value per service: Kcal: 232| Fat: 10 g |Net Crabs: 15 g | Fiber: 6 g | Proteins: 25 g

Ingredients

- Parsley: 1 and 1/2 tablespoon
- 1 can of full-fat coconut milk
- Dill: 1 tablespoon
- 1 clove of chopped garlic
- Basil: 1 and 1/2 tablespoon
- Apple cider vinegar: 2 tablespoons
- Chopped shallots: 2 tablespoons
- Sea salt: 1 teaspoon
- Black pepper
- Chives: 3 tablespoons

Instructions

1. Put the coconut cream in a bowl, leave the coconut water behind.
2. Add four tablespoon of coconut water to coconut cream, mix until creamy.
3. Add garlic, shallots, apple cider vinegar, parsley, chives, dill basil, salt and, black pepper. Mix it and at least left in the fridge for half an hour for flavoring-infusing.
4. Enjoy this sauce over favorite foods.

33. Turmeric-Tahini Dressing

(Ready in about: 15 minutes | Serving: 8-10 | Difficulty level: Easy)

Nutritional value per serving: Kcal: 123 | Fat: 7 g | Net Crabs: 9 g | Fiber: 2 g | Protein: 8 g

Ingredients

- Turmeric powder: 1/2 teaspoon
- Tahini: 1/4 cup
- Olive oil: 2 tablespoons
- Salt and black pepper, to taste
- Lemon juice: 3 tablespoons
- Cayenne pepper: 1/4 teaspoon

Instructions

1. Mix lemon juice, tahini, turmeric, olive oil, 1/4 cup of water, and cayenne till smooth.
2. Add salt and pepper according to your liking.
3. Serve and enjoy.

34. Super Seed Pesto

(Ready in about: 10 minutes | Serving: 8-10 | Difficulty level: Easy)

Nutritional value per serving: Kcal: 127 | Fat: 3g | Net Crabs: 12 g | Protein: 9 g

Ingredients

- Fresh lemon juice: 1 tablespoon
- Hemp seeds: 1/3 cup
- Sea salt: 1/2 teaspoon
- Basil leaves: 2 cups
- Olive oil: 1/4 cup
- Arugula: 1 cup
- Raw pipits: 1/3 cup
- 1 clove of garlic
- Black pepper

Instructions

1. Put all the ingredients into the blender.
2. Pulse until smooth and creamy.
3. Store or enjoy right away.

35. Egg-Free Mayonnaise

(Ready in about: 10 minutes | Serving: 8-10 | Difficulty level: Easy)

Nutritional value per serving: Kcal: 140 | Fat: 14 g | Net Crabs: 10 g | Proteins: 12 g

Ingredients

- Coconut butter: 1/2 cup
- Warm water: 1/2 cup
- Olive oil: 1/4 cup
- 3-4 cloves of garlic
- Unrefined salt: 1/4 teaspoon

Instructions

1. Put the warm water, coconut, garlic cloves, olive oil, pepper, and salt in a mixer.
2. Pulse until combined. Cool it in the fridge and enjoy it.

36. Coconut Butter

(Ready in about: 10 minutes | Serving: 8-10 | Difficulty level: Easy)

Nutritional value: Kcal: 120 | Fat: 15 g | Net Crabs: 9 g | Proteins: 12 g

Ingredients

- Coconut oil: 1 tablespoon
- Unsweetened coconut flakes: 5 ounces.
- Salt, to taste
- Vanilla extract: 1/2 teaspoon

Instructions

1. Put coconut, salt, and all other ingredients in the mixer.
2. Blend until 15 minutes, scrape the bowl in between.
3. It will turn creamy and stick together.
4. Take out in jar and store.

Chapter 7: Anti-Inflammatory Snacks Recipe

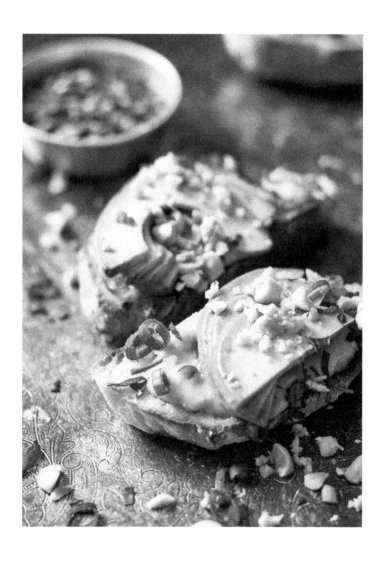

37. Frothy Vanilla Turmeric Orange Juice

(Ready in about: 25 minutes | Serving: 2 | Difficulty level: Easy)

Nutritional value per serving: Kcal: 140 | Fat: 16 g | Net Crabs: 9 g | Proteins: 25 g

Ingredients

- Unsweetened almond milk: 1 cup
- Turmeric: 1/4 teaspoon
- Vanilla extract: 1 teaspoon
- 3 peeled oranges
- Cinnamon: 1/2 teaspoon
- Pepper

Instructions

1. Put all ingredients in the blender.
2. Pulse till smooth.
3. Serve right away.

38. Sweet n' Sour Hibiscus Ginger Gelatin Gummies

(Ready in about: 25 minutes | Serving: 28 | Difficulty level: Hard)

Nutritional value per serving: Kcal: 56 | Fat: 5 g | Net Crabs: 10 g | Proteins: 20 g

Ingredients

- Ginger juice: 1 teaspoon
- Water: 1 cup
- Honey: 1 and 1/2 tablespoon
- Gelatin powder: 2 tablespoons
- Hibiscus flowers cut: 3 tablespoons

Instructions

1. Let the water boil in a pot.
2. Turn off the heat and add flowers of hibiscus.
3. For five minutes, cover and infuse.
4. Take the flowers out.
5. Put the liquid back into the pot, add ginger, honey, and mix.
6. Sprinkle the gelatin over the liquid's surface, then wait for it to melt and mix to gelatin will dissolve.
7. In the silicone mound, pour the mixture.
8. Let it cool down and place in the refrigerator for at least 2 hours.
9. Unmold the gummies, and enjoy.

39. Baked Veggie Turmeric Nuggets

(Ready in about: 35 minutes | Serving: 24 | Difficulty level: Medium)

Nutritional value per serving: Kcal: 60 | Fat: 10 g | Net Crabs: 14 g | Proteins: 20 g

Ingredients

- 1 egg
- Cauliflower florets: 2 cups
- Diced carrots: 1 cup
- Missed garlic: 1 teaspoon
- Broccoli florets: 2 cups
- Ground turmeric: 1 teaspoon
- Black pepper: 1/4 teaspoon
- Almond meal: 1/2 cup
- Salt: 1/4 teaspoon

Instructions

1. Put parchment paper on the baking tray and let the oven pre-heat to 400 °F.
2. In a food processor, add the cauliflower, broccoli, garlic, carrots, sea salt, turmeric, and black pepper. Mix till creamy.
3. Add the egg and almond meal and pulse to mix lightly.
4. Move to a bowl. With your hands, make into discs' shape. Place on the baking sheet.
5. Let it Bake for 15 minutes, and then flip and bake another for 10 minutes. Serve with sauce.

40. Creamy Pineapple Ginger Slaw

(Ready in about: 40 minutes | Serving: 3-4 | Difficulty level: Medium)

Nutritional value per serving: Kcal: 110| Fat: 10 g |Net Crabs: 17 g | Proteins: 20 g

Ingredients

For the creamy ginger sauce

- Red pepper flakes: 1/2 teaspoon
- Soaked cashews: 1 cup
- Lemon juice: 2 tablespoons
- Fresh ginger: 2 inches
- Water: 1/2 cup
- Salt and pepper, to taste

For pineapple slaw

- Cilantro: 1 cup
- Red cabbage: 5 cups
- Red peppers: 4 cups
- Pineapple: 3 cups
- Green cabbage: 5 cups

Instructions

1. Soak cashews overnight.
2. Drain the cashew and add it to a blender along with all other sauce ingredients. Pulse until creamy.
3. In a bowl, add red peppers, cabbage, and pineapple. Add the sauce. Mix it well.
4. Top with cilantro and serve.

41. Turmeric Coconut Flour Muffins

Recipe

(Ready in about: 25 minutes | Serving: 8 | Difficulty level: Medium)

Nutritional value per serving: Kcal: 207 | Fat: 15 g | Net Crabs: 10 g | Proteins: 30 g

Ingredients

- Coconut flour: 3/4 cup, extra 2 tablespoons
- 6 eggs
- Ginger powder: 1/2 teaspoon
- maple syrup: 1/3 cup
- Vanilla extract: 1 teaspoon
- Coconut milk: 1/2 cup
- Baking soda: 1/2 teaspoon
- Salt and pepper: a pinch
- Turmeric: 2 teaspoons

Instructions

1. Let the oven pre-heat to 350 °F.
2. Put milk, eggs, vanilla extract, and maple syrup in a bowl. Mix it. And the eggs until it starts bubbling.
3. Sift the baking soda, coconut flour, ginger powder, baking soda, turmeric, salt, and pepper together in a little bowl. Mix the dry to wet ingredients until fully combined.
4. Put the batter in a muffin tin, dividing equally.
5. Bake for 25 minutes, until the sides are browned slightly.
6. Take muffins from the oven and let them cool.
7. Serve and enjoy.

42. Energy Bites with Golden Turmeric

(Ready in about: 5 hours and 2 minutes | Serving: 8 | Difficulty level: Hard)

Nutritional value per serving: Kcal: 100 | Fat: 7 g | Net Crabs: 7 g | Proteins: 14 g

Ingredients

- Plant-based protein powder: 4-6 tablespoons
- Almond/ coconut butter: 1 cup
- Turmeric: 2 teaspoons
- Maple syrup: 1/2 teaspoon
- Coconut oil: 1 teaspoon
- Coconut flakes: 3/4 cup

Instructions

1. Add coconut flakes (1/2,) nut butter, coconut oil, protein powder, almond butter, maple syrup, and turmeric to a blender.
2. Mix the ingredients at high until well combined.
3. Let the dough rest in the refrigerator to harden for almost 1 hour to 1/2 hour.
4. Take the dough out from the fridge and shape into small balls.
5. Place the balls on parchment paper on a plate, and then move to the fridge for 4 hours.
6. Take out from the refrigerator. Top with coconut flakes and enjoy.

43. Ginger Fried Cabbage and Carrots

(Ready in about: 13 minutes | Serving: 3 | Difficulty level: Medium)

Nutritional value per serving: Kcal: 180 | Fat: 10 g | Net Crabs: 8 g | Proteins: 22 g

Ingredients

- Chopped carrots: 2 cups
- Oil: 2 tablespoons
- 2 cloves of minced garlic
- Coconut aminos: 1 tablespoon
- Cabbage: 4 cups
- Minced ginger: 1 tablespoon
- Apple cider vinegar: 1 tablespoon
- Diced green onion: 1/4 cup

Instructions

1. In a large skillet, heat the oil over medium flame. Add ginger and garlic. Cook for around 1 minute.
2. Add carrots and cabbage. Cook for around 7-8 minutes, until tender.
3. Turn off the heat. Put in vinegar, coconut aminos, almond, green onion. Serve.

Chapter 8: Dessert recipes

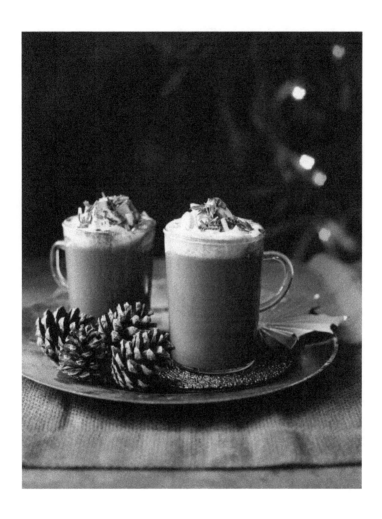

44. Hot Chocolate

(Ready in about: 15 minutes | Serving:2-3 | Difficulty level: Easy)

Nutritional value per service: Kcal: 140 | Fat: 5 g | Net Crabs: 6 g | Proteins: 22 g

Ingredients

- Maca powder: 1 teaspoon
- Non-dairy milk: 2 cups
- Ground turmeric: 1/4 teaspoon
- Honey, to taste
- Raw cacao: 2 tablespoons
- Coconut oil: 1 tablespoon
- Ground cinnamon: 1/2 teaspoon

Instructions

1. Boil the milk.
2. Let it simmer, then add Maca powder, cinnamon, cacao powder, honey, and turmeric and mix well.
3. Then add coconut oil and whisk until it becomes thick.
4. Serve hot.

45. Frozen Blueberry Bites

(Ready in about: 60 minutes | Serving: 16 | Difficulty level: Easy)

Nutritional value per serving: Kcal: 200 | Fat: 8 g | Net Crabs: 0 g | Proteins: 22 g

Ingredients:

- Vanilla yogurt: 8 ounces
- Blueberries: 1 pint
- Lemon juice: 2 teaspoons

Instructions:

1. Mix lemon juice, blueberries, and yogurt in a bowl. Gently mix.
2. Put these yogurt-covered berries on parchment paper and freeze well before serving.

46. Anti-Inflammatory Ginger Gummies

(Ready in about: 60 minutes | Serving: 18 | Difficulty level: Medium)

Nutritional value per serving: Kcal: 157 | Fat: 7 g | Net Crabs: 2.2 g | Proteins: 8 g

Ingredients:

- Non-dairy milk: 1 cup
- Ginger: 2 tablespoons
- Gelatin: 2 packets
- Honey: 2 tablespoons
- Turmeric: 2 tablespoons

Instructions:

1. Add the grated ginger and turmeric in milk. Mix and simmer on low flame for 20 minutes.
2. Strain the milk. Put it back into the pot on low flame. Add gelatin on top, let it bloom, then mix well.
3. Stir in the honey. Pour into the mold.
4. Refrigerate it until hard.
5. Serve cold.

47. Strawberry-Orange Soft Serve, Sorbet, & Popsicle

(Ready in about: 60-70 minutes | Serving: 4-5 | Difficulty level: Easy)

Nutritional value per serving: Kcal: 144 | Fat: 25 g | Net Crabs: 7.5 g | Protein: 26 g

Ingredients

- Frozen strawberries: 454 g
- Orange juice: 1 cup

Instructions

1. Put frozen strawberries in a blender and pulse until all turn to flakes.
2. Add in the orange juice and pulse until smooth frozen puree.
3. Serve right away for soft serve or freeze for sorbet.

48. Gluten-Free Vegan Lemon Cake

(Ready in about: 50 minutes | Serving: 10 | Difficulty level: Hard)

Nutritional value per serving: Kcal: 244 | Fat: 18 g | Net Crabs: 23 g | Protein: 3 g

Ingredients

For the crust

- Maple syrup: 2 tablespoons
- Pecans: 2 and 1/2 cups
- Pitted dates: 1 cup

For the filling

- Crushed pineapple: 1 and 1/2 cup
- Prepared Cauliflower Rice: 3 cups
- Maple syrup: 3/4 cup
- 1 lemon: Its juice
- Vanilla extract: 1/2 teaspoon
- Cinnamon: a pinch
- 3 halved avocados

- Lemon extract: 1/2 teaspoon

For the topping

- Plain coconut yogurt: 1 and 1/2 cup
- Vanilla extract: 1 teaspoon
- Maple syrup: 3 tablespoons

Instructions:

1. Place the ring of 1 inch-inch spring pan on a baking dish with parchment paper.
2. To make the crust: add the pecans in the mixer, pulse until completely chopped up. Add the maple syrup, dates, and pulse for another 1 minute until the mixture gets together.
3. Move the mixture to the baking dish ring and press it to a layer to make the filling. Mix the pineapple, cauliflower rice, avocados, lemon zest, maple syrup, and lemon juice in the mixer — pulse to a very creamy mixture.

4. Add the lemon extract, vanilla extract, cinnamon in the mixer, and mix well. Pour the filling over the crust into the baking tray. Let it freeze overnight or at least for 5 hours.
5. Take out from the freezer and allow to rest for 20 minutes or more. Remove the cake outer ring.
6. To make the topping, mix the vanilla extract, maple syrup, and yogurt in a bowl. Pour over the cake, and serve.

49. Pineapple Upside Down Cake

(Ready in about: 50 minutes | Serving: 7-8 | Difficulty level: Hard)

Nutritional value: per serving: Kcal: 209 | Fat: 9 g | Net Crabs: 9 g | Proteins: 37 g

Ingredients

- Liquid coconut oil: 3 tablespoons
- Almond flour: 1 cup
- Baking powder: 1/2 teaspoon
- 2 eggs
- Vanilla extract: 1 teaspoon
- 15 cherries
- Pineapple: 2 slices
- Raw honey: 5 tablespoons

Instructions

1. Let the oven preheat to 350 °F.
2. Peel and remove the core of the pineapple. In a cake tin, arrange the pineapple slices

and cherries over honey (1 and 1/2 tablespoon.) Bake it for 15 minutes.
3. Mix baking powder with almond flour. In a bowl, mix the eggs well with the remaining honey. Then add the coconut oil and blend well.
4. Take the pan from the oven and dump the batter over the pineapple circles. Go back into the oven and bake for more than 1/2 hour.
5. Take out from the oven and rest for 10 minutes, then switch onto a pan. Serve hot or cold.

50. Lemon Sorbet

(Ready in about: 30 minutes | Serving: 3-4 | Difficulty level: Easy)

Nutritional value per serving: Kcal: 197 | Fat: 17 g | Net Crabs: 10 g | Proteins: 11.6 g

Ingredients

- Honey: 1/2 cup
- Water: 2 cups
- Lemon zest: 2 tablespoons
- Whipped cream, optional
- Lemon juice: 1 and 1/2 cups

Instructions

1. Hours before making, put your ice cream maker tub in the freezer.

2. Put a pot over medium flame, mix the honey, water, lemon zest. Warm it thoroughly.

3. Turn off the heat and then add lemon juice. Mix well. Adjust taste by adding more honey.

4. Move to an airtight jar, and keep it in the refrigerator for at least 2 hours.

5. Move this mixture into a metal pan and let it freeze it for 2 hours. Every 20 minutes, mix to get it airy until it gets to a scoop consistency.

6. Serve and enjoy.

Conclusion

There are certain things you can do to boost your immune system and prevent chronic inflammation. This book provides you 50 recipes to keep a healthy eating plan that can reduce inflammation and improve your whole wellness while eating delicious and natural food.

The diet presented here is based on whole nutrient foods full of antioxidants, one of the elements that reduce levels of free radicals that can lead to inflammation when are out of control. This is the best beginning to stick to good eating habits.

CPSIA information can be obtained
at www.ICGtesting.com
Printed in the USA
BVHW060910250321
603396BV00008B/575